From Motivation to Habit

How Using Your Motivation to Build Habits Will Make You Succeed

Alex Cama

Table of Contents

Chapter 7: What Motivates Different Types of People?

Boosting Student Motivation

Habit Stacking

Get the Students Involved

Motivation for Online Students

How To Motivate Your Online Students

How Do Working Moms Stay Motivated?

Working Moms Are More Productive and Motivated

Motivation

Flexible Goals

Time Management Skills

Moms have good time management skills and are excellent multi-taskers. Multi-tasking is not always great when you have to concentrate on a long project, but many moms seem to be natural at it. You'll find a mom is busy with some serious mental processing while doing physical tasks such as ironing. She's planning shopping and meals for the next day, while at the same time getting clothes ready for the next day. This is a useful skill that many adapt to their work environments as well.

Tips For Working Moms To Stay Motivated

How Business Leaders Stay Motivated

Quick Wins

Opportunities for Transformation

Goal-setting and Commitment

Keeping Teams Motivated

Motivating Children

Introduction

How do you define motivation? It is one of the driving forces of our lives, but it can mean so many different things to different people. Some of us are easily motivated and can sustain our motivation for long periods, while others struggle to get and remain motivated.

If you're motivated and passionate about a project or work that you're doing, you'll often find that you can keep going for hours. The challenge is to sustain motivation during your daily life, and in your career, where you may often need to perform repetitive tasks that tend to become tedious. You might also lose interest if your work is not producing the positive results that you expected, or if it's taking a long time to reach the results.

Passion and Flow

Passion can boost your motivation and focus to the extent that you find yourself entering a "flow" state. The simplest way to describe "Flow" is when you're so focused on a task that nothing else matters. You become absorbed in what you're doing and time seems to speed up or slow down.

A fiction writer might be writing a story with his headphones on, listening to music that becomes part of the background he doesn't focus on and he becomes so immersed in the story and characters he is writing, that he spends an entire day in front of his computer, without noticing.

Passion is important for your success, and you'll be more creative if you're passionate about what you are doing. You'll also have less stress at work and home, if you're passionate and motivated about what you do, most of the time.

Even if you're passionate about what you do, and motivated to make the most of your life in all aspects, there are going to be days and times where you will just feel unmotivated or even ready to give up on what you're doing. For example, the most exciting job will also have mundane tasks which don't interest you. If you're a freelance writer, you might find yourself creating invoices, following up on payments, and doing your taxes.

Building the Habits of Success

The question we attempt to answer in this book is how do you build habits that can sustain your motivation and guarantee your success? We look forward to accompanying you on this important journey.

Chapter 1: What is Motivation?

Described in simple terms, motivation is the force that inspires us to take action in certain aspects of our lives, be it a simple action such as getting a drink because you are thirsty, or something complicated such as quitting your job to start your own business.

Types of Motivation

Motivation allows you to act with commitment to achieve your goals. It is a big field of study with many different psychological theories that describe why people act in certain ways.

Maslow's Hierarchy of Needs

Maslow's hierarchy of needs is a well-known theory of motivation that consists of a pyramid of needs, with the basic needs at the bottom, and the complicated ones at the top.

Maslow's theory states that the lower level needs first have to be satisfied before people can give attention to their needs on the higher levels.

Maslow's hierarchy:

- Physiological - The basics we need to survive such as air, water, food, sleep, and shelter.
- Safety - We need to be protected from threats and dangers.
- Social - We want to belong somewhere, and feel loved.
- Self-esteem - We need respect and recognition.
- Self-actualization - This is the highest level you can aspire to, and includes opportunities for personal development and learning, as well as creative and challenging work.

Maslow's hierarchy forms part of the humanistic theory and suggests that people will only be motivated to meet their advanced needs once they have fulfilled their basic needs. For example, you first need food and shelter, before you can work on self-actualization and fulfilling your potential.

The Incentive Theory of Motivation

The incentive theory of motivation suggests people are motivated to complete certain actions because of rewards. This theory is still relevant today and is often used in the workplace when discussing employee motivation. It is divided into extrinsic and intrinsic motivation.

Extrinsic motivation usually motivates you to perform actions for rewards such as money, a promotion, awards, and other tangible objects. You could also perform certain activities to avoid negative consequences, such as losing your job, because you didn't meet a deadline.

If you're intrinsically motivated, you do something because you find it rewarding, rather than because you expect an external reward, for example, if you are studying a certain subject because you find it interesting, and not because you will be rewarded for doing so. Intrinsic motivation is usually stronger than extrinsic motivation.

The Power of Intrinsic Motivation

This form of motivation can be extremely powerful, as it forms part of your identity and is an ongoing source of motivation.

Extrinsic or external motivation, can't provide you with long-term satisfaction. An easy example is to consider career satisfaction. If you simply go to work because you must go to get your salary, and you get no satisfaction from your job, your productivity and motivation are not going to be great.

The truth is, if you don't have good reasons for why you're doing something, your motivation won't last long.

Improving Your Intrinsic Motivation

There are many ways in which you can become more intrinsically motivated. One of them is to enhance your self-efficacy. If you believe you can achieve something, it's more likely that you will do so.

The term "self-efficacy" was developed by the psychologist, Albert Bandura, and is basically about the beliefs we have about completing a task. If you have high self-efficacy, you will usually be resilient and persevere with completing tasks, even when you face setbacks. However, if you have low self-efficacy for one task, you could still have high self-efficacy for another task.

Volunteering is a great way to improve your intrinsic motivation and also to give back to other people. You can learn new skills and feel good about yourself while staying true to your values such as kindness. Doing something for the joy of it, especially if you also help others, while expecting no reward, will improve your internal motivation.

Your motivation needs to be linked to a purpose that is important to you. You need to understand what drives you, and how your daily activities are contributing to some bigger purpose or goal that motivates you. For example, if you're a teacher, you might be training the leaders of the future.

Don't always wait until you feel like doing things before you do them. Once you start something, you might find that you get into the rhythm and you find your internal motivation to keep going. This often works when it comes to doing exercise. Another way is to set routines and follow them, for example, get up at 6 am to go to the gym. However, this may not work for everyone.

You could also challenge, and set targets for yourself. This could work especially well if you're in a job that doesn't motivate you. Just don't make it too difficult for yourself and make sure you'll be able to reach your goals.

Cultivate a love of learning. If you are a curious person who questions things, you have a reason to keep going and keep working on your goals. You're also much more likely to find your purpose and passion in life if you're always learning new things. Most of the successful and extraordinary people in the world share that trait.

Some of the traits of a learning mentality include listening without judgment, always asking questions, being willing to be wrong, and being able to acknowledge when you don't know something. You should also not worry about failing, as long as you've learned in the process.

The more you learn, the better you will understand yourself and the greater your intrinsic motivation will become, as you will know what you want from life. Live a purposeful life, and go after the goals that are important to you. Unfortunately, many people are chasing goals that they believe are important to them, but their views have unfortunately been influenced by the people around them. You will struggle with motivation if you're not clear about what you want to achieve in life.

Hold yourself accountable for achieving your personal goals. It's easy to give up when you're accountable only to yourself.

Motivation and Habit

While motivation prompts you to get started with something, habits will keep you going until you reach the goals that you have set for yourself.

Habits can also trigger the motivation to start something new. We could also keep doing certain things out of habit.

Starting an action before we feel motivated, could also help us to get things done. Often, when you are already busy with something, repeated actions will give you the motivation to keep going.

The right habits can motivate you or strengthen your motivation.

People who are high achievers, usually stay motivated as a result of the habits they have developed. Successful people usually have the following habits:

- They have goals that are based on their values.
- They tend to focus on the positive, and the progress they've made, instead of failure.
- They know why they're doing something, and their values keep them going.
- They surround themselves with positive and energetic people.
- Some studies have shown that successful people start their mornings with simple habits such as making their beds, making a list of goals for the day, and visualizing the achievement of their goals.
- They also track their progress throughout the day or week.
- They change their routines to learn new skills and look for new experiences. They don't do the same things every day.
- Some successful people join support groups or find accountability partners.
- Successful and highly motivated people are also usually intrinsically motivated and they can learn from others' actions without comparing themselves to them.
- They are open to receiving feedback and learning from positive criticism.
- They are always learning, and willing to learn from their failures.

- They are eager to get out of their comfort zones and don't mind struggling while learning something new.

The Habit of Getting Started

In his book, "Motivation: The Scientific Guide on How to Get and Stay Motivated" author James Clear states you don't need that much motivation once you've already started an action. Clear suggests starting a habit is the most difficult thing to do, and he gives some suggestions as to how you can develop the habit of starting.

Clear suggests that if we have routines that have become habits, this is sufficient to motivate us. It is much easier to start if you have habits for doing exercise, writing, and others. According to Clear, you need to set times for your activities as you will then be more likely to proceed even if you're not motivated.

Chapter 2: What Motivates You?

It's easy to become demotivated, especially when you have a lot on your plate, such as a career, family life, studies, and other commitments. One way to improve your motivation is to find out what you want in life. For many people, their careers give them a sense of purpose and add meaning to their lives.

Finding Your Career Purpose

Some people manage to find a deep sense of purpose by blending their passion and talents to make a deep and meaningful contribution to the world. Is there a way to find your purpose if it's not that obvious to you, or is it just something you find during your life?

Finding your deeper purpose can take time, but you're more likely to stay motivated to reach your long-term goals, once you find them. This is especially true when it comes to your career.

Career Purpose Through Your Side Hustle

A successful side hustle can send your career and personal life in a whole new direction. You may find you have new motivation and purpose where you dreaded working before. The side hustle could even become your new career, which is useful when you have to manage family life as well. However, when you want to manage a new freelance career and a family at the same time, you'll need to develop good habits to keep everything going.

The safest way to start a side hustle is exactly that: as a separate income stream on the side while you still have a full-time job to fall back on if things should go sideways. A side hustle is just an extra job you do outside your full-time job.

Ironically, you may find that a side hustle can boost your motivation for your current job. It might be a case of if there is a deadline in sight for leaving your current toxic job, things just don't seem so bad anymore.

The Motivational and Emotional Benefits of a Side Hustle

Many people have side hustles to make ends meet or to save extra money. It's a great motivational tool as well if you've lost interest in your current job, and you're struggling to keep going. If your job has become tedious and you dread going there every day, a-side hustle project might just be what you need.

Of course, you will still have to do your job as well (at the beginning at least) but a side hustle can help you think more creatively and out of the box, as you have to find ways to make your part-time business a success. It's something to get excited about, and you can push all your passion into this project.

Before you start with your side hustle, you need a vision for your life and career. If you're a busy parent, your to-do list may already be endless. Try to decide what you see your life looking like within the next five years and if you could see your side hustle becoming your full-time business.

Determine how many hours per week you will need to devote to work, and how much family time you'll need. Ask yourself if the side hustle you want to start is truly your passion and if it will let you be more creative. Or are you simply doing it for extra money?

Side hustles can have various emotional and motivational benefits. It can relieve the stress from your day job, and bring you a new sense of happiness and purpose.

Outlet For Creativity

A side hustle can be an outlet for your creativity. This will especially benefit you from an emotional and emotional perspective if you're a creative person who finds yourself stuck in a day job that is extremely structured or involves a lot of administrative work. A creative side hustle will give you an outlet, while you earn money at the same time.

Learning New Skills

You may find that you learn a new set of skills from your part-time job. This is great if you eventually want to change your side hustle into a business, or even just to have new useful skills if you want to apply for another job.

If you're in a conventional job, you usually only learn skills that can be used for that particular job. However, if you have a side hustle, you usually need to broaden your skillset. You often have to do much of the work yourself, such as administration, marketing, or building a website.

A Sense of Purpose

Your side hustle can help you develop a new sense of purpose. Maybe you will realize that your job doesn't satisfy you anymore and that you're just stuck in a comfort zone. You could also learn new skills and go out there and make things happen for yourself with your newfound confidence. You could become successful at a time in your life when you thought you would be stuck in the same job forever.

New Opportunities and Connections

A successful side hustle could lead to new opportunities and connections. You could meet people who open new doors for you; something which wouldn't have happened if you never started your side hustle.

Empowerment and Confidence

Your part-time job can boost your confidence and be a vehicle for personal growth. You may find that you can now interact with business people with confidence, something you could not have done before starting your own business.

You are now important in your own right, and have to make things happen for your business; you're no longer an employee with a job level who has to do as they are told by a boss. You are empowered and you have more authority and control over your own life when you're the one calling the shots.

A Sense of Freedom

A side hustle could also give you a sense of freedom, and a better work-life balance, especially if you manage to turn it into a full-time business.

Financial Stability

A part-time job gives you income stability and helps you diversify your income. You can use the extra money your earn toward your entrepreneurial efforts, or for anything you want that gives your pleasure, such as a luxury holiday. Another financial benefit is that if you lose one client, you won't be left entirely without an income.

A side hustle forces you out of your comfort zone and encourages you to look at life differently. Your new skills and motivation will give you a renewed passion for life.

What Do You Need to Consider When Starting a Side Hustle?

Starting a side hustle can be super exciting, and will boost your motivation to new levels. There are certain things you need to think about, however, before you put all your effort into your side hustle.

Consider the schedule; does it allow you to set your hours? If you want your part-time job to stay that for now, you need one that allows you the flexibility to set your hours.

Decide how much time and effort you can put into your side hustle. If you want to make money quickly and easily, a part-time career as a content writer or blogger might not be for you. If you want to build a long-term business and you're good at writing, it's worth your while to look at blogging, as many bloggers are making huge amounts of money every month.

Make sure you enjoy your side hustle, especially since part of your motivation for starting one, is that you don't enjoy your day job all that much.

Figure out what skills you need to learn to make your part-time job successful, or if you'll be able to use your current skills, for example, if you're a secretary but you feel teaching is your calling, you can do a short course on teaching online and then apply for part-time jobs in this field.

If you're a busy mom and you also want to cut your commute, it makes sense to start your side hustle from home. It might not be practical to have a side-hustle where you have to do a lot of driving around.

It's also essential to decide who is going to run your side-hustle business. Will you work alone, or with your spouse or a friend? If you're going to be running your business with someone else, it's best to draft an agreement.

Habits of Successful Side Hustlers

You need to cultivate good business habits if you want to be successful at reaching the goals of your part-time business. What is known as "good business sense" is often supported by these habits.

Successful side-hustlers usually draw up a plan of some kind before launching their business. A plan doesn't guarantee your success but makes it much more likely that it will happen.

Successful entrepreneurs also tend to stick to the milestones on their plan, and they don't keep putting things off until another day. They meet their goals to determine their progress.

Successful side hustlers are problem solvers and tend to think outside the box. They can usually find novel solutions to problems.

Another important skill is that you must learn the habit of walking away from a venture that is not going to benefit your side hustle. It's essential that you know when it's the right time to walk away from something.

If your business grows, you'll need to learn to hire the right employees and delegate responsibilities. If you like to micromanage every detail, you'll just end up holding your business back and you won't meet your goals.

When you have a new business, accept that perfection is almost impossible to achieve, and at this stage, it's more important to deliver your product or service.

Take things one day at a time and persevere. Learn from your mistakes, like other successful business people had to do. Almost no one is successful from the get-go, they fail, learn from their mistakes, get up and try again.

Healthy Habits That Will Contribute to Your Success

On a more personal level, you also need good health habits if you want to meet all your business goals.

From the start, you need to realize you'll be working more than an eight-hour day. You'll need a lot of energy to keep going, so it's best to avoid sugar as much as you can, even though many people use it as an energy booster. The energy it provides is not sustainable and you will crash, and your productivity will suffer.

Also, make sure you stay hydrated, as this can be a major energy boost. Carry a water bottle with you, and try to drink a certain amount of water every day. You will function better overall if you stay hydrated. Exercise will also increase your energy levels and improve the blood flow to your brain.

Wake up earlier if you want to spend more time working on your business. You can usually work in peace as very few other people are around.

Habits will only make a difference if you do them consistently for some time. You need to set off a chain of habits. If you start by getting up early, you might find you now have time for a habit which you didn't have before.

Chapter 3: Develop a System for Goal Setting

When setting your goals, you might hope you have enough willpower and motivation to achieve them. If you're working towards a specific goal, such as starting your own business or embarking on a new career path, a goal-setting technique could help you set focused, specific goals.

Goal Setting Techniques

There are various goal-setting techniques that you can use to make your life easier.

SMART Goals

SMART goal setting is probably the most popular and widely known goal setting technique. This technique states that your goals should be specific, measurable, achievable/actionable, realistic, and time-bound.

SMART goals can be explained as follows:

- Specific: Your goal needs to be clearly defined. For example, if you want to start a business as a writer, in which niches will you specialize?
- Measurable: You need to be able to measure your success in meeting your goal, e.g. maybe you need to set time limits for certain milestones. You want to earn a certain amount after some months, or you want a certain number of clients.
- Achievable/Actionable: Make sure you can meet your goals with what's currently happening in your life. For example, if you want to find new clients for your business, make sure you can cope with the work you already have.
- Realistic: Make sure you're able to meet a goal. If you're starting a new business, do you have backup cash to keep you going for a few months if you're not making enough money initially?
- Time-bound: Your goal needs a time frame. If you're planning to leave your job to start a new business, decide on when exactly you will do this.
- If the time frame is vague, you may find yourself postponing your goal and never actually achieving it.

SMART goals can also be expanded into SMART(ER) goals.

- Evaluate: At regular time intervals, check that you are making progress on achieving your goal.
- Readjust: Change your goals and plans if necessary. You need to be flexible, for example, if you get assignments that need you to work overtime. Spread your project over a longer period.

The HARD Technique

The HARD technique for goal setting stands for heartfelt, animated, required, and difficult. The letters are widely taken to mean the following:

- Heartfelt: Imagine how proud you would be of learning a new skill, e.g. if you need to learn new computer skills for your freelance writing business. Connect the emotion of pride with your goal, and then use that as motivation for learning.
- Animated: You need to visualize your goal. Imagine what it would feel, smell, sound, or even taste like, and remember that feeling when you think about reaching your goal.
- Required: Connect your goal to something you have to do. If you have to write a blog for your company, try to connect the research to your personal goals, e.g. a blog or website that you want to establish for your own business.
- Difficult: Set a challenging goal for yourself. You'll feel accomplished when you manage to reach it.

WOOP Goals

WOOP goals are useful when you want to get rid of a bad habit.

The letters in WOOP stand for the following:

- Wish: Wish for an exciting goal and attach a positive feeling to it.
- Outcome: Visualize a successful outcome for your goal in vivid detail and think of how you would feel if this should happen.
- Obstacle: Think of what might prevent you from achieving success, or slow you down. For example, if you don't know much about starting your own business and you make mistakes.
- Plan: Work on finding solutions to the obstacles that might interfere with you achieving success. For example, you can find a mentor who can teach you about starting your own business.

Micro Goals

The secret to reaching your main goal is to divide it into smaller sections or pieces (micro-goals). These smaller, achievable goals can play an important role in your ultimate success.

Our serious long-term goals, like losing a lot of weight, writing a book, or buying a house, might soon overwhelm us and we can lose motivation. Usually, we take on too much and we end up quitting because our goals start to seem unachievable. Setting smaller goals or milestones can keep us going on our journey to reaching our main goals.

For example, if you want to build a freelance business, you should set aside time every day to market yourself and find new clients, while doing the work you already have.

You need to be specific with your micro-goals, e.g. I will complete building my business website by the end of the week.

Micro goals help us succeed for the following reasons:

- They increase our motivation as we can see some results. You're more likely to continue pursuing something if you can see progress, e.g. if you write 1 000 words a day of a 100 000 word novel. If you have these manageable goals, you will be less likely to quit before reaching your main goal.
- Meeting your micro-goals can increase your overall happiness, and boost your brain's dopamine production. This will increase your positive thinking that will go a long way in helping you reach your main goal. We often stop going after our goals as a result of low self-esteem, and negative thinking.
- Micro goals also reduce long-term stress, as you tend to focus on consistent effort, and not your big, scary goal.
- You'll also have a greater sense of control if you have various small goals since you can change some of these goals if you realize something isn't working.

How to Make Your Micro Goals Work

First, decide on your long-term goals, and set completion dates for them. Then you can work backward to work out your micro-goals, and by when you would need to complete certain tasks to reach your main goals.

Write a daily list of the micro goals you aim to accomplish. You will stay on track if you know exactly what you need to accomplish every day.

Consider what you need to do at the present moment to accomplish your daily goals. If you take mindful, small actions throughout the day, they will all contribute to helping you achieve your long-term goals.

Measure your daily micro-goals regularly, to determine if you are still on track to meeting your long-term goal. Also, make sure that your daily goals are manageable. It's easy to become demotivated if you put too much pressure on yourself.

Setting Goals According To Your Personality Type

You might find that certain goal-setting techniques don't work for you, and this could be because you are trying to do something that goes against your personality type. Your personality type can also influence how motivated you are to work on certain goals.

There are three main personality types when it comes to the planning stage of goal setting:

1. The analytical type of personality enjoys writing and planning their goals until the smallest detail. The SMART technique of goal setting works well for this personality type.

2. The intuitive type of personality doesn't like to write down and plan their goals. If you're this type of personality and you force yourself to write goals down, you might start to feel overwhelmed and start procrastinating. This type of personality will go all out of a goal if they're convinced the goal is reasonable and achievable. The SMART method can help this personality type figure out if a goal is reasonable for him or her.

3. The hybrid personality is at times analytical about their goals but can be more intuitive about other goals.

When it comes to executing goals, type A and type B personalities will also have a different approach.

Competitive A types will go after their goals with everything they have, even if the goal is somewhat overwhelming. Type B personalities are more likely to be successful when they approach their goals milestone by milestone.

Different personalities will also approach the completion stage of reaching the goal differently.

- There are those people who are super excited and inspired to get started on achieving their goals, but then get bored and might abandon their goal once they get over the excitement.

  If you're this type of personality, you need to find a way to keep your goals interesting, by raising the bar of whatever it is you want to achieve. Also delegate the aspects of the goal that don't interest you, if you're able to do so.

- Some people can achieve a goal, whether it remains interesting to them, or not. However, they might find it difficult to change course and waste time working towards a goal that is no longer relevant.

The Four Tendencies Framework

Gretchen Rubin, an American author, and researcher created the Four Tendencies Framework. According to Rubin, there are four major personality types--upholder, obliger, questioner, and rebel--that are motivated by different things. Her theory is that people encounter inner and outer expectations in life. How you respond to these expectations provides insight into your personality.

Rubin describes the four personality types and how they respond to goals, as follows:

1. The Upholder meets inner and outer expectations. This type of person is goal-oriented and loves following rules. They always seem to meet deadlines and are highly conscientious people. They thrive on structure and plan rigorously to make themselves and everyone else as happy as possible. On the downside, they can insist on following rigid rules that aren't needed and they get upset when others aren't as consistent with keeping commitments.

2. A Questioner meets inner expectations while resisting outer expectations. Questioners are focused, and they are devoted to logic and research. They are efficient

people and tend to pick and choose rules that seem to make sense to them. Questioners can overanalyze and tend to have difficulty making decisions. They find it difficult to let go if their questions haven't been answered.

3. An Obliger resists inner expectations but meets outer expectations. They are selfless people, and mostly put others before themselves. They will drop everything to help other people and they're usually productive workers and team players. On the downside, they might get burned out from focusing so much on other people, and neglecting their self-care. They are often overextended and unable to meet their personal goals.

4. Rebels resist inner and outer expectations. They enjoy autonomy and will speak up for themselves and others. They thrive well when they can be independent and deal well with a lack of structure and spontaneity. On the downside, they can find it difficult to relax, and they could be uncooperative or unresponsive when they are asked to do something.

If you fall into one of these personality types, you should adjust your goal-setting techniques to align more with your strengths.

How to Meet Your Goals

To be able to set goals that you can achieve, you must also be in touch with what you want in life. There is no use in setting goals to achieve something that you don't want in the first place.

Your goal setting must not be influenced by family expectations, pressure from your family or friends, or past goals which you couldn't achieve. For example, if you decide on a career or studies to pursue, focus on what you want to achieve in life and where your interests lie. Otherwise, you might never complete your studies, or you won't last long in your career. Many people wake up in mid-life to find they've made the wrong decision when it comes to their career and qualifications.

Set goals that are important to you on an emotional level. You will see that the emotional reward after completing a goal such as winning a race, can encourage you to set more goals.

Your goals can include other people, but should not depend on them for success. For example, you will study with a partner to get good exam results. However, you can still study alone and get good marks, even if your study buddy doesn't show up all the time.

A Personality Test Can Help You Set Career Goals

If you're not sure what career goals to set, or you want to change your career, a personality test could help you on your way.

Enneagram

The Enneagram test has become especially popular in the workplace in recent years.

The Enneagram test offers in-depth insight into your personality and can be used for greater self-discovery and self-awareness. The test uncovers patterns of behavior that motivate us to behave in certain ways. Once you understand what motivates you to behave in a certain way, you can develop new habits and change your behavior. The Enneagram allows you to take responsibility for your personal growth, as you can set new long-term goals.

The Enneagram test can have important benefits for individuals, teams, and organizations as a whole.

Benefits for individuals:

- It can help you set achievable goals, and increase your productivity.
- It can assist you with building confidence.
- Help you understand your behaviors that are the result of your core motivations.
- It helps you increase your compassion for yourself and others.
- It creates authentic leaders and helps them make more impact.

Benefits for teams:

- It can help teams make sense of conflict and other issues.

- It helps you understand your team members better, and encourages you to act in a more tolerant manner towards them.
- Improves productivity and working relationships in general.
- Improves business procedure.

Benefits for organizations:

- Reduces toxic organizational politics
- Increases organizational productivity and creativity
- Reduces fear of change
- Improves leadership and enables culture change
- Assists with employee development

You can view the world based on one of the nine ways of your enneagram core motivations. These motivations are broken down into nine core fears and nine core desires.

The core desires for the different types are as follows:

- Type 1: Being Good/Right
- Type 2: Being Wanted/Loved
- Type 3: Being Valuable/Admired
- Type 4: Being Authentic/Finding Meaning
- Type 5: Being Competent/Capable
- Type 6: Being Secure/Supported
- Type 7: Being Satisfied/Content
- Type 8: Being Independent/To Protect Themselves
- Type 9: Being at Peace/Being Harmonious

The core fears for the different types are as follows:

- Type 1: Being Bad/Wrong
- Type 2: Being Unwanted/Unloveable
- Type 3: Not Being Valued/Admired
- Type 4: Not Having Significance/Meaning

- Type 5: Being Invaded/Overwhelmed
- Type 6: Having No Support/Security
- Type 7: Being Deprived/Emotional Pain
- Type 8: Being Controlled/Weak
- Type 9: Being Separated

Myers-Briggs Type Indicator (MTBI)

This personality test is based on Jung's theory of psychological types and can help you with choosing a field of study and career planning.

The test focus on the following things:

- How you perceive the world, you're either an extrovert who enjoys the company of other people or an introvert who prefers your own company.
- It also looks at how you process information. Do you sense (basic information) or do you add additional information (intuition)?
- Are you a logical and consistent thinker or do you consider the people and circumstances (feeling) surrounding a situation?
- When you process information that you receive from the outside world, do you judge quickly, or are you open to new information (perceiving)?

The test has 16 personality types that are indicated as codes of four letters. It is a simple multiple-choice questionnaire that you can take at mbtionline.com. You select the answers that are the best fit for you, and there are no correct or incorrect answers.

You can get your results in the form of a profile report via the website.

The following is an overview of the personality types:

1. The ESTP enjoys social interaction, reasoning and logic.
2. The ESTJ is a leader who believes in traditional values. This personality is always happy to take the lead and to provide guidance to other people.
3. The ENTJ personality is a natural leader and tends to view obstacles as opportunities to excel.
4. INTP - This personality is good at reading people, and thrives in creative environments.
5. ISFJ - This personality is kind-hearted and always ready to help other people.
6. ENTP - This rare personality is an extrovert who doesn't always thrive in social situations. They are rational, logical, and objective people.
7. ISTP - This personality is introverted, enjoys meeting people, and can be spontaneous and fun.
8. ISTJ - This type is serious, reserved, and hardworking. They value tradition.
9. INFJ - These creative idealists are usually imaginative and have fantastic ideas. Other people find them strange and amusing, because of the unique way they look at the world.
10. INTJ - This quiet personality is a true introvert, and needs to get away from other people to recharge.
11. ENFJs are charismatic people-pleasers, who are good at connecting with people from all backgrounds.
12. ISTP - This rational, and logical personality type, can be spontaneous and tend to hide its true characteristics from other people.
13. The ESFJ is your stereotypical extrovert and loves being in the spotlight and interacting with others.

14. ESFP - This born entertainer is lively, and fun, with good people skills.
15. INFP - This quiet and reserved personality enjoys making sense of the world by spending time alone.
16. ENFP - This personality is a leader, who doesn't care about the status quo. They're good at thinking outside the box.

Chapter 4: Overcoming Self-Sabotage

Sometimes your fears and negative self-talk can hold you back. If you have habits and beliefs that are demotivating you, you must confront them. You can't force yourself to be motivated, and you need to be kind to yourself. Talk to yourself as you would to a friend—with kindness and respect. You may find that you need to overcome the negative ways of motivation that you learned during your childhood.

Limiting Self-Beliefs

It can be scary and difficult to make a big lifestyle change such as quitting your job to start your own business. You must change your way of thinking and overcome your habit of self-sabotage when setting goals.

Your fears might stop you from setting effective goals and your way of thinking might sabotage you in the following ways.

Lack of Self-Belief

If your self-belief is not strong enough, it will be difficult to form habits for sustained motivation.

You don't believe you can succeed, and you're not sure what you want out of life.

You don't even want to bother to improve yourself and learn new skills, because you firmly believe you'll never reach your goals.

These negative patterns could have been formed in childhood, for example, if you had overly critical and controlling parents. You'll have to confront your negative perceptions of yourself before you can make any progress.

Unrealistic Expectations

If you're not successful immediately, you lose interest and motivation.

If you're a perfectionist, you might expect yourself to be successful all the time. You're scared of stress and expect things to go smoothly all the time. You don't want to ask others for help, as you want them to think you're perfect.

If you want to remain motivated, however, it's essential that you set realistic goals, and expect that you'll have to deal with stressful events on your journey. It's impossible to avoid stress, but your life will be so much better if you know how to deal with it.

Fear of Disapproval

You might fear that other people like your friends or family might disapprove of your desire to change and that they won't take your new goals seriously. You might have failed in the past, and now you fear you won't have their support to try again. It might then seem like a better idea to avoid any effort and trouble, and just remain the way you are. However, you will regret this, when you look back on your life.

Fear of Disappointment and Uncertainty

You were motivated and psyched up in the past to do something major, and then you failed, or only reached some of your goals. Now you'd rather stay in your comfort zone, as you're afraid the same thing is going to happen again.

To be able to make progress, you're going to have to confront this fear. If you want to succeed at a project, it's important to have a growth mentality and learn from your past mistakes. Maybe you just didn't plan enough or you gave up too soon. If you've failed once, it doesn't mean you'll fail again.

Those who see their failures as learning opportunities are usually able to recover more quickly and are also more motivated to set goals for sustained success.

Comparing Ourselves With Others

If you compare yourselves with others, you'll end up angry and disappointed. It may appear to you that others don't struggle and succeed easily, but they often have challenges you don't know about, and their problems are different from your own. Only focus on your own goals and keep your nose to the grindstone. In this way, you will be successful sooner, without being distracted by the activities and successes of others.

Inflexibility and Fear of Uncertainty

It is hard to adapt to disruptions to your goals if you're too inflexible. If you struggle to deal with uncertainty, you'll be more likely to stay in your comfort zone and avoid changes. If you want to motivate yourself and set new goals, you will first have to deal with this mindset, and change your behavior, before you'll be able to make real changes.

Procrastinating When Starting Out

If you set your sights too high when starting on a new venture, you might find yourself procrastinating around starting your business, instead of jumping in there and getting things done. It's not always a great idea to compare yourself with others who've been successful in the same field, as it may make you feel that you don't have the necessary resources to start at all.

You now convince yourself there are many new skills you need to learn first or people you have to meet before you can even think of starting your business.

However, everything doesn't have to be perfect for you to start a venture or business. Sometimes the best option is just to start, and then improve on something as you go along. For example, you can waste a lot of time, and money, planning and building the "perfect" website for your freelance business. In reality, you can start with a few simple pages on WordPress, and improve them as your business grows. The idea is just to start something and to get your name out there.

The excuse that you first need to learn more, or organize more, could become a crutch that leads to you not doing anything to get started. Waiting for the ultimate strategy or idea turns into a way to get yourself out of doing hard work.

Overcoming Limiting Self-Beliefs

Now that you've pointed out the limiting beliefs that are holding you back from being motivated and setting goals, you need to find ways to overcome them. You might have to keep going with nagging negative thoughts at the back of your mind, at least for a while.

Try these tips to help you overcome limiting beliefs:

- Learn to plan, and follow through with your plans. Challenge your negative thinking and forge ahead, with your plans. If you plan as well as possible, you're also less likely to be disappointed.

- Learn to deal with frustration and disappointment. You're strong enough to deal with it, and you don't want to regret the things you didn't do, 10 years from now.
- If you fear stress, planning can also help you alleviate this problem, so that you have more time to focus on your goals. Also manage how many tasks you take on, to help you manage your stress levels. This can also help you prevent burnout. Also, minimize your stress by trying to cut down on the time you spend on social media and other activities that are just a waste of time. Learn to ask for help when you need it.
- Perfectionism when setting your goals is also a type of self-sabotage. Starting new projects can seem daunting, and it's also a good way to waste time and to avoid starting for as long as possible. Sometimes you just have to start a venture and make mistakes, while learning, as part of the journey.
- When you're comparing yourself to others, keep in mind that you don't know how hard they worked or how many setbacks they suffered on the road to success. Typically, it's only the success stories that make it to social media.
- If you want to stay motivated on your journey, you're going to have to accept that life is chaotic and most of the time it won't follow your rules. When things go wrong, you can accept the challenge, and try to find creative solutions to problems.
- Try to be flexible and open-minded in all areas of your life. This will also help your brain develop new pathways when things go wrong and you have to solve problems.
- If you're going to do something new, don't be too impatient when you set your goals, and pace yourself. Set milestones that are easy to reach before you get to

the main goals. Reaching small steps can make you feel that you are progressing, and give you a sense of achievement.

Fear Goals

Sometimes, if you find yourself getting discouraged after setting your goals, it helps to run towards your fears. "Fear" goals can keep you going, as often what we are most afraid of doing, is what we should be doing. The hard choices can often lead us to the greatest success.

When you're afraid of doing something, it sometimes helps to visualize your fears and put your thoughts down on paper.

The following exercises encourage you to analyze your thinking, which could help you make a decision:

- Draw columns on a piece of paper, and then write down what inaction will cost you in 5, 10, and 15 years.

  For example, you want to leave your job to start a business, but you're scared to give up your guaranteed income, and you're afraid you won't meet your personal financial goals if your income is uncertain for a time. However, even though your job guarantees you an income, you find it tedious and you can't use your core skills, which you will be able to use, should you start your own business. Your job is also stressful, it's taking a toll on your health and is harming your relationship with your family.

  After you have carefully considered all the facts surrounding your current job and your potential business, write down where you think you'll be after the different periods if you remain in your job and you never start a business. This exercise should already show you why we often regret the things we never did, later in our lives.

- Another useful exercise you can do on paper is to write down the worst outcomes you can see for your decisions in one column, write in the second column next to it what could have been done to have prevented the negative outcome, and in a third column write how you would repair the damage of a negative outcome.

  For example, if you start your business, but you find after some time that you're not making enough money to pay your bills. In the second column, you can write your ideas on how this could have been prevented, e.g. you could have spent more time and effort on marketing.

  In the third column, indicate what you can do to mitigate the situation, e.g. you can take a part-time job to improve your cash flow, while you work harder on marketing your business and getting new clients.

- Also, consider the benefits of attempting to do something, or being partially successful. What have you learned from attempting to start a business and what can you do better? You can use this knowledge to set you on the right track, to decide on new goals.

How To Motivate Yourself After Failure

One of the most difficult things to do in life is to motivate yourself to get back after a massive failure and to try again. Many people would regard themselves as permanent losers, or tell themselves that they will never be able to achieve something. However, the truth is that those who win big in life, are simply losers who didn't give up, learned from their mistakes, and kept on trying.

Failure doesn't have to mean the end of your journey; it could just be another step you need to take on the way to success.

Some people find it helps if they implement new strategies to achieve their goals after they fail at reaching their objectives. Failure is a setback, but one that can teach us important lessons. It's even possible that you'll be more successful eventually, as a result of what you've learned from your failures. Famous successful people like Elon Musk failed many times before finally achieving success.

Try to deal with your failure as positively as possible. It's a negative and miserable situation, but see what you can learn from it, to prevent future failures. The best way to deal with failure is to regard it as preparation for future success.

Don't let your failure define you. If you failed at a work project, look for ways to overcome the problems you experienced, so that they don't happen in the future. Accept your failure and move on from there.

Failure will teach you things that you can't learn from your parents, partners, or other people in your life. You can identify your strengths and weaknesses and develop some strategies to improve.

Failure can help you become more organized. Don't procrastinate about your failure, by agonizing about what you could have done better. Use this opportunity to plan for future success. Don't worry about what others think about you.

Find inspiration to recover from your failure and gain motivation for the road ahead. Look for a motivator on the internet and find one who relates to your current situation and failure. Also, turn to supportive family and friends, as it's good to have a shoulder to cry on and they can also motivate you to continue moving forward.

In the case of a business failure, re-evaluate your processes in detail and plan your services going forward. Look in detail at the mistakes that happened, and why some of your services weren't a success.

Get Past Fear-Based Decision Making

If you want to get past failure and ultimately succeed, you need to be able to push past making fear-based decisions, as this decision could often lead to you making no decisions at all. You need to do the things that are important to you and don't be afraid of other people's judgment or opinions.

If you're one of those people who worries excessively about other peoples' opinions, remember that most people don't care if you fail or if you're a success. The world is full of people, and you're not going to be on the minds of that many people. Chase your dreams, even if you've already failed more than once, without worrying too much about what other people think.

You need to get past thoughts telling you that you're destined to fail. You might be destined to succeed, and it's just going to take you some time to get where you want to be. If you've failed once, or even more than once, it doesn't mean you will fail again.

Remember that the only real failure is taking no action at all. Many people let themselves be held back by their feelings of uncertainty and fear. If you've taken the brave decision to do something, this already separates you from most other people. You're the one person who's decided to do something and pushed through with it, which puts you on the road to success.

Plan For Failure

The other way to overcome failure is to plan for it. It takes hard work, mastering essential skills, and planning to be successful, but if you want to reduce your stress and increase the chances of your long-term stress, you need to plan for failure as well.

One of the reasons people lose motivation and can't keep up with their habits to reach their goals is because they haven't planned for failure. If you plan for failure it doesn't mean you plan to fail, but that you know how you will get your efforts back on track if things shouldn't work out.

If you've come to realize that individual failures won't have that much impact on your long-term success, you will be able to come back more easily from failure.

Chasing Your Dreams In Middle-Age

It takes courage and motivation to chase your dreams if you're already middle-aged, if you're employed in a cushy corporate job, it's the middle of a pandemic, and you have kids to look after. But there's never a right or wrong time to chase your dreams, even if you feel you're swopping one kind of stress for another.

If you're already middle-aged with responsibilities, you may think it's not a good time to start a business, but the truth is, there's never going to be a better time than now. Whatever age you are, you're going to find excuses to keep putting it off. You're going to find ways to talk yourself out of it, so you need to get past the first obstacle of simply starting.

Talk to your family about what is important to you, start planning, and get your show on the road. Quitting a job is never a small decision and it could potentially have a huge financial impact on your family.

Do the research and get support by talking to other business people who are experts in their fields. They could give you useful advice on what business software you need to get healthcare insurance for your family.

Be creative with creating income streams while you're in the process of starting your business. If your business is can't fully support you yet, see if you can find other opportunities for making an income, like working part-time, or looking for online opportunities. You could help out friends or family, and even discover other talents you didn't know you had, which could come in handy in your business.

Motivational Tips for Starting a Business

Chasing your dream and working hard for what you want, is also a good example for your children. You can show them that there's more to life and that they should go after what they want.

While it can be difficult to get the motivation to chase your dreams, you must take charge and do what you think is right at that time, even if you're scared.

You must learn what mistakes to avoid from crushing your dreams, while you're chasing them.

Don't allow yourself to be overwhelmed by discouragement. No one ever said chasing your dreams, starting a business, etc. was going to be an easy road. Even if you don't reach your goals at first, you will learn a lot and you could even find new opportunities in the process of reaching for your dreams.

If you come across speed bumps while chasing your dream, change your course.

If you find yourself in a bad situation, don't live in denial. You need to deal with the obstacles you're facing and work toward changing them. Believe in yourself and keep on going.

It's not worth your while to dwell on a painful past, as you'll use all your energy to worry, and you'll be afraid to make decisions. Don't be afraid of making decisions because of past bad experiences, as you'll keep yourself back from using opportunities.

Don't procrastinate, as you're most likely letting opportunities pass you by. Just get things done when they're supposed to be done, as you can never get wasted time back.

It's vital not to neglect your health, mentally or physically, while you chase your dreams. Eat as well as possible, and take time to exercise. If you get sick your motivation will drop, and you will have to take a break from working toward your goals.

Go out there and make things happen for yourself; don't wait for other people to come to you. Many doors will be closed to you, but you need to find the open ones, or even go in through the window. Change the course of your plan, if you think there are other ways in which you can be successful.

You will be judged by other people for the life you're living, how you look, and many other things. Don't take it personally, and be proud of your journey. The judgment all has to do with their fears and insecurities.

Keep Chasing Your Dreams When Life Is Overwhelming

If your life is stressful and difficult, it can be difficult to focus on reaching your goals and dreams. You need to have a clear vision of what exactly you're chasing. If you're not sure what you want, you need to spend some time alone writing done your goals. Then put them up where you can see them every day. You will be reminded of what you are working towards. Also remember, dreams take time and effort.

There will be times that life gets in the way of your dreams. You'll have family issues or fall sick. You need a solid plan of action for those times when your life gets too overwhelming to give your full attention to whatever it is, you're chasing.

The fact is you need to motivate yourself to find the time to go after your dreams. You may think you don't have time to work toward your dreams such as starting a business or writing a book, but the fact is you do have the time. You can find the time to watch several episodes of a TV series, go to sports events or concerts, hang out with your friends or be lazy and do nothing. It's simply a matter of priorities. You usually manage to make time for whatever is important to you.

You may need to make adjustments such as waking up earlier, cutting out TV, and spending less time with your friends. If you're serious about a dream such as starting a business, you need to make sure you put enough time into it.

Keep going and plow ahead. If you want to achieve success, giving up should not even be an option for you. Fail, make mistakes, and make adjustments, but never give up when you are working towards achieving your goals.

Boost yourself with the knowledge that will help you achieve your dream. Read when you have time, listen to podcasts and watch YouTube videos to learn as much as possible about the particular dream you're chasing. This will help you stay motivated, even when you're not working directly on achieving your dream. In a sense, you should "live" your dream as much as possible, in every aspect of your life.

To help yourself reach your dream, set deadlines and smaller milestones for yourself. For example, if you want to write a book, set various deadlines for yourself by when you will have your chapters and characters outlined.

Ignore any self-doubt you may be feeling, as this will just cause your motivation to crash.

Allow for changes and learn to adapt, as you chase your dreams. If something should disrupt your plans, it will be better to readjust than to quit. If you're flexible and open to adjustments, you'll be motivated to chase your dreams when life gets overwhelming. It may take some focus, but it's possible to find the motivation to go after your dreams when life gets overwhelming.

Chapter 5: Procrastination

Procrastination is a major form of self-sabotage and deserves a chapter on its own. It involves putting off important work or other matters until the very last minute or right before the deadline.

You then have little time left to do a good job and cause yourself unnecessary stress. Some people prefer to work in this way, but it's always best to avoid rushing to get a job done if you can do so.

How to Manage Procrastination

Procrastination can be caused by underlying feelings of anxiety, such as a fear of failure. There are ways you can make work and projects more manageable for yourself, such as breaking projects into more manageable, smaller pieces, setting limits on the time you take to begin a project, and you can work towards completing tasks as quickly as possible. You could also reward yourself after completing sections of a task.

Why Do You Procrastinate?

If you need to know the causes of your procrastination, you need to analyze the situations in which you're not managing to complete your work:

- Do you have a problem with time management, and you're always running late?
- If you don't find a project interesting, or it's not relevant to your values, you might struggle to complete it.
- If you're not sure what exactly is expected of you, it might also be difficult to get started.
- If you're a perfectionist and hard on yourself, you might also find it hard to start a new project. This is even

more difficult if you're anxious about other people evaluating your work.

- You might also be anxious if you're venturing into a new career or field, as you're not sure how well you will do.
- If you feel you're unable to manage the tasks - you didn't have training or you lack the skills, you may also struggle to get started.
- You could be underestimating the work involved in completing a task, or overestimating your abilities and the time you will need to complete the task. You may think you have a better understanding of the subject matter than you have.
- You may think short repeated delays are harmless, such as spending five minutes on Facebook, instead of working or completing a term paper. However, before you know it, you end up spending your entire evening on social media, and you get no work done.
- Do you say you're committed to getting something done, but then you never end up doing it? For example, you decline invitations to parties, because you say you need to study, but you never do.
- Maybe you spend a lot of time on getting part of a task perfect, such as the introduction of an essay, but you don't get time to move on to the rest of the task.
- You could struggle to make up your mind between choices, for example, you spend so much time researching different term topics, that you don't have enough time to write the actual paper.

Practical Ways to Overcome Procrastination

- Make sure that you know exactly what is needed to complete a task within a certain time frame.
- Also, be reasonable in what you expect from yourself. If your expectations are too perfectionistic, you may end up sabotaging yourself.
- If you don't want to spend too much time on a task, admit this to yourself, and don't feel guilty.
- Plan your projects appropriately, and break them up into smaller segments where possible.
- Also plan for relaxation, as you will be able to complete your work more successfully if you have downtime.
- Monitor your projects and if you're meeting your time commitments.
- If you have fears, like a fear of failure, making mistakes, or even a fear of success, you must deal with them. Certain fears, such as a fear of success, because you believe you don't deserve it, may indicate deeper issues that need to be resolved as they might keep on preventing you from achieving your goals. Addressing these fears will go a long way in resolving your procrastination habit.
- It's also important to recognize the signs that you're heading for procrastination. If you start thinking that you'll leave something for later, or you don't feel like doing something now, don't give in to the urge to stop, but keep on working as long as possible.
- If you tend to procrastinate, it's also best to eliminate distractions as far as possible. Turn off all distractions such as social media or television for a certain time, and just focus on the task you need to complete.

- Reward yourself after you complete a task. Do something you enjoy, such as watching your favorite television show, or attending a concert.

Chapter 6: Getting Started and Building Momentum

As discussed before, momentum will sometimes come to you only after you start a new behavior. Sometimes action, even though you don't feel like it, will encourage momentum.

You may have experienced this when working on a project, sometimes it is overwhelming to think about even the beginning, but the closer to the ending you get, the more motivated you become.

For example, if you're a writer, it will mostly not work to stare at your blank page, waiting for inspiration, as you could then take a long time to get started and you won't meet your deadlines. It's often best just to get started and the ideas will flow as you write.

Habits and Rituals

Some people have simple, almost mindless rituals to help them get started on more complex tasks. It's as if starting with a simple step in the morning can set off a series of events, which lead to their higher levels of cognitive functioning being triggered; almost like a chain reaction.

It seems if you focus on a simple ritual, the next steps can be almost automatic, even if motivation and decision-making don't form part of the process. Your brain doesn't have to expend energy thinking about your first steps. You set a pattern of steps in motion and the rest of the sequence will follow.

We can use the ritual of getting children ready for school in the morning as an example. You are not motivated to get up, but you do so and start the same steps that you follow every day. You prepare the school uniforms, wake up the children, prepare their lunch boxes, give them breakfast and take them to school. Possibly your brain will only start functioning once you get home and you have to get started with your work.

The idea of the ritual is that it relieves you of the burden of having to make decisions when you're brain doesn't feel up to it. You don't have to take any decisions on what to do or how to get started. Many people can't get moving, simply because they can't make up their minds on how to get started.

Once you've started with something, you have to motivate yourself to keep going and reach your milestones or goals.

The Goldilocks Rule

In his book on motivation, Atomic Habits, James Clear refers to the "Goldilocks Rule". This refers to a way of retaining motivation at work and in life, by working on tasks that are difficult, but manageable for someone of your abilities. For example, if you play chess against a small child, you'll get bored, but if you should play against one of the chess masters, you will lose motivation as they will easily defeat you.

What you should be doing, is playing against someone who has an equal ability to yourself.

The game will be of manageable difficulty to you, as you have a good chance of winning, but you also have to focus and try hard. This is a good example of the Goldilocks Rule that states that humans experience their highest level of motivation when they're working on tasks on the edge of their current abilities.

Along with working on tasks at the right level of difficulty to keep you motivated, it's also essential to measure your progress on an ongoing basis. Seeing yourself make progress, or receiving positive feedback, can be very motivating.

A combination of these factors can cause you to experience "flow" when you are immersed in doing something. Also known as being "in the zone" flow is the mental state you're in when you lose track of the rest of the world.

It seems these are the two simple steps for long-term motivation - doing tasks at a just manageable level of difficulty while measuring your progress and receiving immediate feedback, if possible.

When Your Motivation Plunges

Sometimes, you have to show your mind who's in charge. Or you might have to show the devil and angel on your shoulder, whispering suggestions into your ears, who is the boss of your destiny. The devil is whispering that you're tired and you need to give up. The angel is telling you, that you'll feel good about yourself once you've completed the project and reached your goals. She whispers that you can finish the task. It's finally up to you to decide which option you want to choose.

Remember that most of your discomforts are only temporary. We create a lot of our stress, as lives are easier now than they've ever been in human history.

You feel proud of your good work once you have completed something, but remember that it takes effort and work to get the desired result. It's sometimes difficult to start something, but it's always worth finishing, even if you could only do an average job on that particular day. It's vital to remember that accomplishments always take hard work and effort.

If you think about it, life is often about having to decide to be disciplined and keep on working to reach your goals, such as studying to pass your exams, or taking the easy way and giving up. Our everyday life decisions are often a battle between the easy and hard ways.

Also, keep in mind, if you're working on a project that is part of your life's purpose and that you're passionate about, you're less likely to become demotivated. This will also be different from person to person. For example, I might not regard writing content or fiction as hard work, as I am a creative person and that is my passion in life. However, if this does not come naturally to you, and you rather be out there working with people, you might regard it as draining, hard work.

Motivation and Creativity in Life and Work

Creative people work out of the desire to create order in their world, and it is a bonus to get rewarded or applauded for their work. There is a strong link between internal motivation and creativity.

Creativity adds meaning to our lives. A creative accomplishment rarely happens overnight, but is usually the culmination of years of internal motivation and hard work.

Edward de Bono's concept of lateral thinking or thinking outside of the box encourages creative thinking in business and the classroom. The following are ideas for creative problems solving:

- Try reverse thinking. See something in the opposite way of how we normally would, and garner more creative ideas.
- Question your assumptions about things, so that you don't fall into a rut.
- Suspend your judgment on an idea that does not seem attractive at first glance.
- Try to see how a situation is similar to one that is different from it.
- Find the dominant idea in a book, conversation, or presentation.

Creative employees with good problem-solving skills do most of the highly valued work in the modern economy. Their jobs are to plan, analyze, create innovative products and manage your company. Creative workers who are motivated are more innovative and productive than those who aren't. They deliver the highest quality work and are always looking for better ways to complete their projects. It's therefore in companies' best interests to keep these employees motivated. When creative employees don't have the drive to excel at their work, quality will plummet, which can lead to financial losses for companies.

It's entirely possible to improve the quality of creative employees' output, by encouraging their intrinsic motivation. Creative employees want to do meaningful work of their own choice, at which they can establish their competence and where they will see themselves making progress.

Creative workers with sufficient internal motivation will perform better on projects than employees who receive substantial external motivation such as monetary rewards.

It's interesting to note that many big and successful creative projects are taking place without monetary rewards. A good example is the IT industry, where people take part in open-source software projects and contribute to the code, for the sake of learning and building a useful product.

In general, employees with sufficient internal motivation are more satisfied with their jobs, they're less susceptible to negative stress and they have better career development.

Encouraging Creativity at Work

There is no straightforward answer to the question of how to motivate creative workers. It simply depends on the people and the type of work done in your organization. Some might be motivated by extra challenges, and others may want more independence. It's finally up to you to get to know your employees well and to find out what works for them. If you know the intrinsic factors that motivate different employees, you can use these in your organization's favor.

Achievable Goals

Work should have achievable goals, as that will add to their feeling of making progress. Project goals should be attainable, but also challenging to the extent that employees can feel they have managed to achieve something when they finish a task. Reward employees once they reach a goal, but the reward will be more motivating if it's in the form of respect and recognition, rather than a tangible reward.

Another way is to get your employees to determine their own goals. This will increase their accountability and it will also make the work more meaningful to them if they have a choice. One method is to let them set objectives and key results that are visible to the entire company, as all the employees can then see how the various teams are making progress and improving.

Give Them a Choice

It's also an intrinsic motivator for employees to be able to make choices around their work tasks. Creative workers want to feel they can control their work projects and control what they are involved with. It will motivate them if you include them in decision-making and give them a chance to make an impact on their day-to-day work.

Google has a great way to make creative workers part of the decision-making processes at the company. They have the

Google Ideas website where employees can submit ideas, and their proposals for new products and processes.

Google also has 20% time, an initiative where creative workers can use 20% of their work time for projects that are outside their regular tasks, but which could benefit the company. This provides even more opportunities for employees to be creative and innovative. Google has managed to get important new products from this initiative, namely Gmail and AdSense. The initiative aims to show employees that their initiative and ideas are appreciated.

Motivation and Meaning

Employees are also more inclined to be intrinsically motivated if they feel their work has meaning.

Encourage your employees to care about the reasons for their day-to-day work. The company needs to engage about the purpose and the significance of the work it does.

You should also recruit employees whose values align with your company's values. Employees need to do work where they feel they can make a difference so that they can experience the company as being inspirational and motivational.

Supporting Learning

Learning and building their competence will motivate employees, and they must receive learning support. If your employees are interested in something that will possibly be useful to the company in the future, it makes sense that you encourage their learning and even pay for their studies. Lifelong learning and education are important in today's ever-changing business world.

Respect

Google has another creative and unique way to show respect to its employees through its weekly TGIF meetings. During these meetings, top management takes any type of questions from employees, nothing is off-limits.

Chapter 7: What Motivates Different Types of People?

Some people manage to stay motivated and can reach their goals under extremely stressful circumstances. This is especially true for students, many of who have been faced to turn to online learning during the Covid-19 pandemic, working moms whose lives became even more hectic during the pandemic, and business leaders.

Boosting Student Motivation

It may be hard for students to build good learning habits, especially if they are not internally motivated by what they're doing.

Some students may be mediocre in most of their subjects, and then suddenly excel in a specific area, as they are motivated to do so. If you're a student, or you teach students, take note that students must discover what keeps them going throughout the day and what their interests are.

If you know your students' interests, you can try to make it a part of your lessons together. For example, if you know some students enjoy cooking you can boost their motivation by making it part of lessons such as maths (fractions) or even writing classes.

You should try to learn as much as possible about your students and what their interests are, as this will make it easier for you to help them with motivation and goal setting. Motivation is the key aspect that will influence their performance.

Habit Stacking

Habit stacking also works well to encourage motivation in students. If we help students learn in manageable chunks, they're much more likely to build skills that will lead to them achieving their larger goals. Teaching English as a foreign language class is a good example of training that already follows this format. The lessons are usually broken up into phases and start with a fun introduction to a new subject, before then moving on to a section where students learn the vocabulary they will need for a lesson. Before moving on to the core of the lesson, the teacher will first test the students' knowledge of the vocabulary through a series of tasks, some of which are performed with a partner. After the main section of the lesson, there is also a closing or a "Cooler" in which the learning that happened during the lesson, is summarized.

Get the Students Involved

Students may also get demotivated if they don't feel enough responsibility for what they're doing and teachers make also the decisions when it comes to running classes. It's essential to keep students interested and involved. Get them to work in groups and bring their material and resources that they can present to the class.

Motivation for Online Students

The advantage of the rapidly expanding online learning environment is that students can learn new skills and get qualifications from their location, without having to go through the expense or hassle of securing transport, and possibly traveling for an extended period before reaching their universities or schools.

Student motivation has become an important topic during the ongoing Covid-19 pandemic where classes were increasingly forced to move online, especially during the height of the various infection waves.

How To Motivate Your Online Students

Motivation is vital when it comes to online learning. Students lost motivation when they felt isolated due to the reduced social interaction and lack of face-to-face classes.

Recent studies determined that online participation plays a significant role in boosting the intrinsic motivation of online learners, as they tend to lose motivation when they are left on their own. The students still prefer engaging environments where they can interact with others, the feedback is more immediate and there is a collaboration between students.

As a teacher, there are several techniques you can use to keep your students motivated online.

Try to give feedback as timeously as possible, as delayed feedback in an online learning environment may contribute to the students' feeling of isolation and may demotivate them even further.

There are various options and programs you can use to give feedback almost instantly in the online environment:

- You can have virtual feedback sessions via Zoom during which you also discuss important issues.
- With the program, BookWidgets, you can design activities with built-in feedback.
- Some programs like Jing allow you to provide video feedback with screen captions.

As a tutor or teacher, you can also motivate your students through your enthusiasm. This is even more important when students are studying online. They will observe your passion for the subject you're teaching, and if you don't appear interested, they will also lose motivation. Try to have a lively and entertaining online discussion and link the material back to their everyday lives.

It's important to use a variety of instructional methods. Your students will all have different learning personalities. Some will be visual learners, and the information will have to be displayed to them colorfully and interestingly. Others may learn better through listening, and they will benefit from interesting class discussions and lectures.

You will have to make sure your online learning material includes as many options as possible for different learning personalities. Make sure you include videos, discussion boards, textual information, PowerPoint presentations, and more.

Study resources should always be easily accessible. Students will lose motivation if they have to struggle to find material or the material doesn't download properly. Google Drive should work well for the resources you want to upload. Also, provide students with guidance on where else on the web they can find study and reading materials.

Provide your students with concrete examples and do your best to link theory to practice. Your online students will stay motivated if they believe what they're learning will help them achieve their professional and personal goals.

Organization and planning are essential to maintain student motivation and interest in the online classroom. You don't have as much room for improvisation as in the real-life classroom, and you need to plan as well as you can for a smooth and effective learning process.

If you want your online students to remain motivated, you need to help them improve their autonomy. It will go a long way in helping them stay motivated if you help them get control over their educational process.

You can help your students be more independent in the following ways:

- Create a calendar of assignments and make the study materials available to the students, so that they can plan their long-term studies.
- Allow your students to set their long-term goals and take ownership of their learning at the beginning of the course.

Students will also be more motivated if they can keep track of their progress and learning. A good way is to request them to keep a portfolio of their work from their first work to whatever assignment they completed last. Ask them to reflect on their learning after each assignment they complete.

If you're teaching adult students, also keep in mind that they will be more motivated to learn if they're treated with respect as unique individuals with interests and lives of their own. If they feel you're on their side as a coach, they will feel more comfortable contributing to classes. With adult students especially, you need to strengthen their internal motivation so that they are less dependent on you for their learning.

How Do Working Moms Stay Motivated?

When it comes to motivation, we can learn a lot from working moms who normally have a lot of responsibilities they have to juggle at the same time, every day. It's kids, household, and career—and with the Covid-19 pandemic, this situation became even more intense, as homeschooling children were added to the mix.

There are many reasons a working mom could lose motivation; fatigue being one of the main ones. Their goals could also become unattainable or delayed when life becomes too busy with the additional demands children place on a woman.

Yet, most moms continue to thrive in their careers, and even as entrepreneurs. So how do they motivate themselves, especially when they're exhausted and feeling like they're running on empty?

As discussed elsewhere in this book, a lot of it has to do with time management and planning.

Working Moms Are More Productive and Motivated

Research has found that working moms are often more motivated and productive than other employees, even though they have more responsibilities and stress. Working mothers are also successful entrepreneurs, even those with small children.

Many working mothers say becoming a mom has contributed to their career success. They've become more innovative at work, and they're better managers and business owners than before they had children. Much of it seems to have to do with gaining better time management skills.

Motivation

Many moms are more motivated at work since they know they have to manage their time between their job and kids. This allows them to develop habits to get the work done, as they lose precious time with their children if they have to work overtime.

On the whole, working mothers also have a greater sense of purpose, as they are happy to follow their passion.

Flexible Goals

Once you become a mom, you realize it's nearly impossible to create a perfect household where everything runs smoothly. However, working moms can use the experience they gain at work to make their households run more smoothly, and vice versa. Many do set SMART goals, and evaluate the outcomes, to make their lives run better. If they set up a plan to run their households, it needs to be flexible, and be for different scenarios.

Working moms are more focused on their goals, as they have to prioritize their busy days. They are also more aware of their strengths and weaknesses, and what they need to work on to succeed at work and home.

Time Management Skills

Moms have good time management skills and are excellent multi-taskers. Multi-tasking is not always great when you have to concentrate on a long project, but many moms seem to be natural at it. You'll find a mom is busy with some serious mental processing while doing physical tasks such as ironing. She's planning shopping and meals for the next day, while at the same time getting clothes ready for the next day. This is a useful skill that many adapt to their work environments as well.
Working moms are also better and directing conversations and waste less time to get the information they need.

When it comes to time management, working moms are excellent at prioritizing. You quickly learn to let things go if you identify them as not being a priority. The time you work is spent away from your family, so you need to focus to get the most important jobs done.

You can also get better at working with people as your empathy develops. You get more flexible and make the best of every situation. You also develop leadership skills.

Tips For Working Moms To Stay Motivated

If you're a mom who struggles to get motivated, there are some simple tips to help you get through the days:

- Connect with other parents and share helpful advice. Their kids don't have to be the same age as yours, as those with more experience might be able to share helpful advice with you. Those with kids at the same life stage as yours will also be able to share advice and commiserate with you.
- Support other working moms at your office, even if it's only in small ways. Share your knowledge with your colleague who has just returned from maternity leave.
- Take some time for yourself and implement some self-care routines. If you're physically and mentally healthy, you'll be more motivated at home, and work. The time can be difficult to find, but try to plan for it, even if you only get to do it occasionally. Also savor small, quiet moments, like you have during your child's naptime, or in the car before going to work. Find time for exercise, even if you have kids exercising with you.
- Make a list of everything you have already accomplished. This will remind you that you're still the same accomplished and motivated person, who has goals and dreams to achieve.

How Business Leaders Stay Motivated

Senior business leaders can also teach us a thing or two about staying motivated in adverse circumstances. Working in a world that has been hard-hit by the Covid-19 pandemic during the last two years, they have found themselves working in increasingly difficult economic circumstances.

So how do they do it? Or are they just more strong-willed and confident than the rest of us, and that is how they've managed to get their positions in the first place?

Many organizations find themselves in crisis, and one of the first steps leadership can take is to accept that it will be temporary. Most leaders know that this situation is not unique and businesses have found themselves in tough situations before. So how do business leaders continue to motivate themselves and their employees during these challenging times?

Quick Wins

Business leaders tend to focus on the most vital part of tasks that will go towards solving whatever crisis there might be in their company. Good business leaders are careful not to assign more than their employees can handle, as this will decrease the morale of their staff.

They know the quick wins will keep the staff going when they are faced with a long uphill battle to restore confidence in their business. Small wins are motivational as they signal to the brain that progress is taking place, and that bigger success could be just around the corner.

An excellent business leader will highlight every success that is achieved during a difficult time. It gives employees hope that things are changing for the better and that they're almost at the end of a hard time.

Opportunities for Transformation

Talented leaders will realize that a crisis provides them with the opportunity to make changes in their workforce. This should motivate them to introduce new energy into their company. They need to be able to see the positive side of the crisis, and how it can help them make their company or brand more competitive.

Goal-setting and Commitment

Leaders might aim high, and set goals that aren't easily achievable. They will keep striving for their goals and won't let negative thoughts deter them.

Good leaders are also open to change and will adjust their values with time. They're flexible and able to deal with uncertainties. However, they won't forget their original goals and plans.

Successful business leaders will also reflect on their progress and see where they can improve. They will always measure how far they are from reaching their goals.

Great business leaders also have a high level of commitment, which is critical to their success. They are committed to the wellbeing of their company and its employees, and this is what keeps them focused when they don't feel motivated.

Keeping Teams Motivated

Besides staying motivated and inspiring themselves during tough times, leaders also have to keep their teams and employees motivated.

- Successful leaders usually have a good understanding of their employees and of what is important to them. Good leaders understand that their employees all come from different backgrounds. They also do their best to build good relationships with their employees.
- Some leaders will go the extra mile to show their employees, that they view them as part of the family, and not only as workers. They will send personalized birthday messages, condolence messages to an employee who has lost a loved one, or other congratulatory messages.
- Senior leaders who excel value the input their employees make to keep the company moving forward. They always listen to their employees as they know that employees lose motivation and feel ostracized by the company if they feel misunderstood.
- Great leaders know that their company's success depends on ongoing teamwork. They realize they can't claim the company's success for themselves, and that they will fail if they do that.
- Leaders realize it's also necessary to provide their employees with extrinsic motivation from time to time, such as a bonus or extra time off.
- Excellent leaders also can share the vision of their company with their employees and motivate them to buy into it. Employees will follow a leader or CEO who has a clear vision for their company.

Motivating Children

Children are internally motivated from a young age to learn as much as possible about the world around them. Adults can facilitate this process by encouraging their natural curiosity and desire to learn.

Parents and teachers need to provide positive motivation during learning and development.

You can do the following to motivate children during the learning process:

- Let your baby explore new objects and events. You will find they look away from objects that are too familiar to them, and are no longer interesting. They will also look away from new objects that they find too complex. Look at what your baby finds interesting, and try to build on these interests.
- Provide your infants with the opportunity to interact with new objects. Let them do what interests them, and learn from this.
- Encourage your children to play and explore. Play intrinsically motivates children to learn. It provides them with an opportunity to experience new things and they can learn from others. It can also reduce stress and help them form social bonds. Play is essential for their development.
- Even though children can learn from digital media, and many educational computer-based applications have

been designed for children, they still need social interaction with their peers and adults, for learning to be effective.

- You can motivate your children to work toward achievable goals. They need to be challenged when they do something, but at the same time success must also be possible. They will lose motivation if the task is too easy, but also if it is too difficult to achieve. Some video games use this principle of learning effectively, by increasing the level of challenge based on a child's performance. When you adopt a challenge for a child based on their capabilities, also provide them with regular feedback on their performance.
- Kids are usually more motivated when they are left to do things for themselves to a certain extent and they can choose to do tasks that they find interesting. They're more likely to stay engaged and motivated when they can choose their projects and can make decisions about how they want to do things.
- Give rewards to children only when it's really necessary. If they're suddenly rewarded for something they usually enjoy doing, going forward they may want to only do it when they know they will be rewarded for doing so. This will reduce their internal motivation. Rather let them use their natural intrinsic motivation and curiosity to work toward achievable goals, than promising them rewards for their efforts.
- Praise your children for their efforts to achieve something and not necessarily the grade or award they received, as they might develop a performance orientation. The danger is that they could be motivated to work hard for more rewards, but they might not want to be involved in activities that they're not good at, as they might fear negative evaluation. You need to help

your children see failure as an opportunity to learn from their mistakes. They will then be more likely to believe that they will be able to achieve their goals.

- Many children try to push boundaries when they become teenagers. This is a natural desire to learn new things and become more independent. Teenagers are motivated by the approval of their peers and it may be tempting for them to be risk-takers and break boundaries. However, teens who have parental support and an open relationship with their parents are less likely to become involved in risk-taking behavior such as substance abuse.

Homework and Learning at Home

Do you struggle to get your kids to do their homework, or to be enthusiastic about doing the extra reading? Children also need to be motivated to learn outside the classroom.

If you want them to be enthusiastic about learning at home, you can't always tell them what to do, how to write, etc. as they will become bored. You need to give them more control so that they can decide what and how they want to learn.

It's essential to create a reading atmosphere at home so that your children can improve their communication and vocabulary skills. Reading at home will improve their confidence to read in class.

Try to determine your child's strenghts and what their interests are. Buy books for your children that will encourage them to excel at their favorite subjects, such as math books.

Create an open communication channel between yourself and your child. They should be able to share with you, if they have challenges with learning, or if they have any concerns.

Listen to their suggestions, and don't show disapproval, otherwise they may lose interest in studying.

Try to make learning as fun as possible for your children, by adding games or whatever else they enjoy. Allow them to study in different rooms of the house, if they become bored of their study room.

Help your children discover their unique style of learning, and let them try out different styles. They will feel more motivated to continue learning if they're free to use their style.

Have flexible study times. Allow your child to continue playing if they are involved in an interesting game, especially if they're younger. Young children also learn a lot from playing.

Why Intrinsic Motivation Is Essential for Children's Learning

Internal motivation, or children's own desire to learn, is essential for their development. Having this type of motivation makes them want to improve themselves and gain more knowledge.

Most children only go to school to have to, so the challenge is to increase their internal motivation so that they will want to learn for the sake of gaining knowledge.

Evaluation can influence children's learning. If we focus more on grades than feedback about the learning process, there is the danger that they will only learn when they can get good grades, and they will lose interest in subjects where they can't perform as well.

The problem with education that focuses mainly on grades is that the students tend to focus less on quality learning and don't involve themselves in learning in a meaningful way.

They then lose motivation, and school turns into a burden for them. That's why we must encourage children to become involved in mastering a subject and not to only focus on passing or failing. It's vital to focus more on feedback than grades in the classroom, to keep children motivated and engaged with the learning process.

Another way to encourage intrinsic motivation is to get children involved in creating learning material. You can also ask them to participate in evaluation and grading.

Teachers can also motivate children by getting them to reflect on the study process itself, and their strengths and weaknesses.

Students with intrinsic motivation will have the best learning experience. To truly gain from the experience of learning, they need to feel that they want to face the challenge of learning.

Motivating Children With Learning Difficulties

Staying motivated while learning can be even more difficult for children who struggle while learning. Many of these children's self-esteem gets a knock when they keep on trying to do something well, but it ends up still not being good enough. That's also where grades can play a role in demotivating children. They might lose the desire to keep pushing themselves to learn and improve.

Children who struggle with certain things at school regularly have negative experiences. If a child struggles with a certain subject, he might stop turning in his homework, as he knows he will have many incorrect answers, and he fears the teacher's reaction. These types of experiences can cause kids to lose motivation and feel like they're not good enough.

The question is what will help kids who struggle at school stay motivated and keep pushing themselves to improve? How will they stay motivated even when they have to face serious challenges?

Rewards can play a role, even if they are simple, such as praise and positive feedback from a teacher, or a good grade.

Getting internal motivation is even more difficult for kids who struggle, as they progress slower than their peers, and they face more challenges and setbacks. For example, they might stop studying if they keep on doing badly in tests. They might get defeated to the point that they start expecting bad outcomes for most of their tests. This may discourage them to the extent that they start avoiding other challenges.

You can help your child with learning difficulties stay motivated at school. Help them a little bit at the start of a big project so that they can experience some success and positive moments. This will boost their motivation and self-esteem to keep going on the project. For example, you can help your child with the outline for his project, and this might help him to engage better with the writing process, and build his confidence. Hopefully, he will feel successful while researching and writing his paper, and this will give him confidence and motivation for his next assignment.

Focus more on effort when it comes to your child's studies and not so much on the outcome. Praise them for a good grade, but also ask them how they studied for the test. Did they use specific techniques? Also, do this if they didn't do that well in the test because then they might discover a new approach for studying for the next test.

Encourage your child to develop a "growth mindset" from a young age. This will motivate your child to always believe he can improve with practice. If your child falls into the trap of a fixed mindset, he'll believe that he can never be good at something which he is not naturally good at.

If your child fails at something, focus on moving forward and the steps to take so that he can succeed the next time.

Some children lose the motivation to try new things if they fail at their projects. Try to get them out of their comfort zones as having new experiences is the only way that they can learn what their passions and their strengths are.

That's why they need to try new hobbies or learn new skills. Remind them that everyone struggles at first when learning a new skill.

Recognize small successes even if they failed in the bigger scheme of things. Tell them they were good team players, etc.

Motivation and the Elderly

Many people tend to lose motivation as they age. You may start to feel that your time is passing and that you're just a burden to your family. Your health may not be great, and you start developing all kinds of aches and pains that make you not want to get out of bed in the mornings.

Elderly people who once used to be good sportspeople may find the physical aspects of aging particularly difficult. They may have old injuries that start to bother them.

Some also struggle with the psychological aspects of their declining physical appearance. A woman who has been praised for her beauty her entire life may start to withdraw from society if she is embarrassed by her aging physical appearance.

Our linear view of life is part of the reason why we tend to lose our motivation and "lust for life" as we get older. For example, after you leave school, and university, you build a career and marry the love of your life with who you raise a few children. After you retire and your children no longer need you to support them, there's not much point for you to keep on existing.

The fact that we live in a youth-driven media culture also doesn't help us stay motivated as we age.

Staying Involved and Finding a Purpose

One way to stay motivated as you age is to stay engaged with the world and to keep on contributing as you can. You need to stay involved and you will keep feeling as if you're making a difference. You're never too old to make a difference in the world and to keep on learning new things.

Reach out to the younger generation and learn from them about the world they live in. In turn, they can gain useful skills and knowledge from you.

Many people find aging traumatic and try to cling to their youth. When you get older, you need to find a new useful purpose in life, even if it's something small from day today. The more you wallow in self-pity, the harder it will get to be engaged with your family and friends, as well as the world around you.

Motivating the Elderly People in Your Life

If you want to motivate and support the elderly people in your life, you'll have to stay positive and kind. They may have developed a negative mindset as a result of health challenges they have to face daily. If you're worried about their motivation, you should discuss their situation with their healthcare practitioners.

Medication could also be affecting their behavior, and there is the possibility that they could be suffering from Depression. Depression is especially likely if they suffer from diseases such as heart disease, dementia, or stroke. Their medical practitioners should be able to prescribe the correct medicine for any illness they may be suffering from.

You can also ask their doctor for advice on how you can help your elderly relatives be more motivated, and lead a more active lifestyle that will improve their mental and physical health.

In addition, have discussions with your elderly relatives about what is bothering them. They could be depressed because there are certain things they can't do anymore, such as driving. Acknowledge their feelings and offer them support.

If they've already lost a spouse, this may also cause them to feel isolated. Try to arrange visitors or engagements for them that would require engagement. Do simple things such as taking them out for coffee, or simply chatting for a while.

Set a few minor goals for each week to get them to engage more, for example, to go for a short walk in the neighborhood once a week. Before you know it, they could be going a few times a week. No one is too old to set some goals for themselves, and with a little creativity, anything is possible.

If you're a caregiver for an elderly person, try also not to enable their inactivity by doing everything for them. If you do things for them that they could still be doing for themselves, you're just enabling their inactivity, and you end up doing more harm than good. They'll get the message that their unable to do things for themselves, and they will stop learning and growing--it becomes a self-fulfilling prophecy.

Older people should also be encouraged to learn technology to stay in touch with the world around them. It can also help them improve their interpersonal relationships. Some elderly people might feel anxious, and that they're too old to learn new technology.

The elderly can benefit from learning online social technology like email, social media sites, online video calls, and chatting, as well as smartphones. This can also help them stay in touch with their children if they live far away from their kids.

Also, encourage older adults to stay as fit as possible. This can help them stay healthier for longer, and also improve their energy levels. They don't need a schedule of heavy exercise, even taking the stairs or short ten-minute walks will help to boost their energy and fitness. Swimming is a great exercise for older people.

Older people might also benefit from doing volunteer work, as this will help them use their time in a useful way, and they also get to give back to the community, which will make them feel good about themselves. There are even many opportunities to volunteer online, for example, as a teacher or tutor. Volunteering can also get them interacting with other people, and out of the house.

Chapter 8: When Motivation Is Not Needed to Perform

It's nearly impossible to be motivated all the time, no matter what you're working on. Even if you have a fun and exciting job, there are going to be days that you're not going to feel like showing up. You will have off days when you'll simply have no energy.

You can develop routines and habits that keep you performing even on your off days.

The Motivational Routine

Like some sportspeople have pre-game routines, you can develop routines to put you in the best mental state to get you going. By the time you've finished your routine, you should be ready to do whatever it is you need to do.

A good motivational routine needs to be simple so that your brain doesn't have to use too much energy to think about it too much, especially if you're going to be doing it when you get up first thing in the morning. Sometimes you could be in an autopilot state. For example, when you get up in the morning and you walk to the kitchen and make coffee. After this, you do other actions such as putting on your clothes, brushing your teeth, and then walking to your computer to start working.

You could have a routine where you start writing, by putting on earphones and selecting a song; you could even start with your same favorite song every day.

The most important thing is to start. You'll create your motivation by performing a sequence of simple actions.

The idea is just to start with your simple routine, not thinking about what needs to come next. Start with the simple steps and go from there. For example, if you're going to work at creative writing, just turn on your computer, put your earphones on, and then the music that normally motivates you to write. You'll even find that certain songs motivate you to write certain scenes or about certain characters.

Most of these simple "pre-game" routines should include movement, as it's difficult to think yourself into being motivated. If you're moving around, it's a lot more likely that you'll get energized and become engaged. Your routine should gradually include more movement, as your motivation will build with your physical movement.

Another important thing to note with establishing a routine is that you need to follow the same pattern every time. You always need to perform the same series of events before doing a specific task. The routine then becomes so much a part of your performance, that by doing the routine, you get pulled into the right mental state for performing. Eventually, you don't need the motivation to start something at all, but only your routine.

This routine becomes a reminder or trigger that pushes you into doing what you need to do, even if you're not motivated to do it.

If you have to make too many decisions when you're not motivated, you'll just end up quitting, so you need your routine to let you know what you need to do next. You don't have to make any decisions and you just follow the pattern.

Your routine will allow you to train yourself for excellence. The habits that you perform daily will become your identity, which will allow you to become a person who doesn't need to be motivated to perform.

You must perform your routine every time before you do something, as it becomes a good habit and you will also experience positive feelings every time you perform this routine.

This is the difference between becoming successful and staying where you are. If you only work when you feel motivated, it's unlikely that you'll reach your goals or achieve great success. Your routines, which will help you gain good habits, will help you achieve success in the long term.

The Secret to Creating Lasting Habits

If you want to create new and lasting habits, you first have to create a new identity for yourself. Your habits are based on your current identity, and it's subconsciously based on the person you believe you are.

So, to change your behavior, and subsequently your habits for the long term, you need to see yourself in a new light.

If you want real, long-lasting change, your goals need to focus on establishing a new identity first, before you focus on outcomes.

Most people chase outcomes and results before they look at identity, so they're doing it back to front.

Before you do anything else, you need to consider your self-image, how you see the world and how you judge yourself and others. If you start by focusing on the goals you want to achieve, you're creating outcome-based habits, whereas you need to create identity-based habits.

You need to decide on what type of person you want to be, and then start with small changes. Consider your principles and values.

For example, you decide you want to become a better writer, with the hope of pursuing writing as a career. You want to become the type of person who writes 2,000 words a day. A small win in this direction would be to write a few paragraphs every day for some time.

You can do all kinds of activities to motivate yourself, but ultimately if you become the person you want to be, you don't have to rely on motivation to help you reach your goals.

If you manage to build identity-based habits you'll get the best results.

Planning Implementation

Planning and writing down your intentions, will also more likely get you to follow through on doing something. It seems that for some people, having a plan works better than being motivated. A plan helps you turn your initial desire to do something, into action in the real world.

Time and location are essential for implementing your intentions. These implementation intentions help us keep to our goals, whether it's writing down the time when you have a doctor's appointment to writing down that you have to study, going to bed early, and other habits that you want to adopt.

People who have a plan on exactly when and where they will start a new habit, are much more likely to follow through with it. If you find yourself unable to change your habits, it might be that you did not figure out the basic details. We might decide that we will eat healthier, but we never decide on the specifics of when and where this is supposed to happen.

If you leave it up to chance that you might feel motivated or remember to do something, it is most likely not going to happen. Your problem might simply be a lack of clarity and that you're not sure when and where to take action.

If you have an implementation intention, you don't have to wait for motivation, but simply follow your plan.

You need to have a specific time and location so that if you repeat your actions enough times, you will get the urge to keep on doing them.

If you plan where and when you will do something, your environment will trigger your behavior and not your motivation level. If you want to achieve your goals, don't rely on motivation alone, as it often doesn't lead to consistent action. Plan how and when you're going to execute your goals.

Conclusion

Motivation is one of the driving forces of leading a successful life, but it can be a challenge to find and sustain motivation at different times of our lives. If you find your true passion, motivation may come easily. However, it also becomes harder to stay motivated as we get older. This book also provides you with tips on how you can help your elderly relatives retain their lust for life, avoid depression and stay motivated for the future.

Even if we're passionate about what we do, there will be times when we will struggle to find motivation and to remain motivated. There are going to be days when you simply don't feel like showing up, whether it is at work, your business, or in your personal life. During these times, you will have to rely on the habits and routines that you have developed, to keep you going even on your off days.

Eventually, you might find that your "pre-game" routines become so automatic, that you hardly even have days where you feel demotivated any longer. As these routines and habits automatically kick you into gear, your performance in your business/work and personal life will soar. You will have no problem in reaching your goals in any aspect of your life, and you will achieve the success that you have never believed was possible, before reading this book.

We have enjoyed walking this journey with you, and we believe that you will continue to grow and evolve if you use the tips mentioned in this book. Keep on believing in yourself and reaching for new heights. Only you can ultimately find the motivation within yourself that you need to achieve success.

References

"5 Steps to Start Your First Side Hustle | SkillsYouNeed." *Www.skillsyouneed.com*, www.skillsyouneed.com/rhubarb/start-side-hustle.html. Accessed 20 Feb. 2022.

7 EFFICIENT Goal Setting Methods Based on Your Personality Type. 16 Nov. 2019, frankdaemon.com/goal-setting-methods-on-personality-types/. Accessed 20 Feb. 2022.

"21 Quotes That'll Inspire You to Finally Start a Side Hustle This Year." *Thought Catalog*, 25 Feb. 2018, thoughtcatalog.com/ryan-robinson/2018/02/21-quotes-thatll-inspire-you-to-finally-start-a-side-hustle-this-year/. Accessed 20 Feb. 2022.

"Achieve Your Goals by Understanding Your Personality Type." *All Things Admin*, 13 Nov. 2014, www.allthingsadmin.com/goals-understanding-personality-type/.

arlene. "Motivation vs Habit." *In Goode Health*, 25 Feb. 2017, ingoodehealth.com/2017/02/motivation-vs-habit/. Accessed 20 Feb. 2022.

"Best 7 Strategies to Increase Student Motivation Online." *BookWidgets Blog*, 2 Jan. 2019, www.bookwidgets.com/blog/2019/01/best-7-strategies-to-increase-student-motivation-online.

Buckley, Dylan. "9 Types of Motivation That Make It Possible to Reach Your Dreams." *Lifehack*, Lifehack, 11 May 2012, www.lifehack.org/articles/productivity/6-types-of-motivation-explained.html.

Cherry, Kendra. "Motivation: Psychological Factors That Guide Behavior." *Verywell Mind*, Verywell Mind, 27

Apr. 2020, www.verywellmind.com/what-is-motivation-2795378.

"Top Tips for Overcoming Procrastination." *Verywell Mind*, 19 July 2020, www.verywellmind.com/tips-for-overcoming-procrastination-2795714.

Clear, James. "5 Useful Reminders for When You Want to Give Up." *James Clear*, 9 June 2015, jamesclear.com/giving-up.

CPCC, Stephanie Huston. "5 Ways to Figure out Your Purpose and Change the World." *The Startup*, 17 June 2018, medium.com/swlh/5-steps-to-finding-your-hustle-165c39726b67. Accessed 20 Feb. 2022.

Johnson, Genola. "Steps to Finding Your Purposeful Side Hustle." *Medium*, 4 July 2018, gebjohnson096.medium.com/steps-to-finding-your-purposeful-side-hustle-4f5036bfc68c. Accessed 20 Feb. 2022.

"Key Habits You Need for Your Side Hustle to Thrive." *Habit Stacker*, 16 Aug. 2020, thehabitstacker.com/key-habits-you-need-for-your-side-hustle-to-thrive/. Accessed 20 Feb. 2022.

Marinoff, Evelyn. "Why Is Internal Motivation so Powerful (and How to Find It)." *Lifehack*, Lifehack, 8 July 2019, www.lifehack.org/839224/internal-motivation.

Merit Morikawa. "Motivating Creativity - the Why and How of Intrinsic Motivation." *Viima.com*, Viima Solutions Oy, 24 Jan. 2017, www.viima.com/blog/motivating-creativity-the-why-and-how-of-intrinsic-motivation.

"Motivation and Habit - TPW179." *The Productive Woman*, 28 Feb. 2018, theproductivewoman.com/motivation-and-habit-tpw-179/#:~:text=Motivation%20%28as%20in%20a%20reason%29%20can%20help%20us. Accessed 20 Feb. 2022.

"Overcoming Procrastination | Counseling and Psychological Services (CAPS)." *Www.brown.edu*, www.brown.edu/campus-life/support/counseling-and-psychological-services/index.php?q=overcoming-procrastination. Accessed 20 Feb. 2022.

Santora, Jacinda. "What Is a Side Hustle (+ Best Practices for a Successful One)." *Influencer Marketing Hub*, 22 Jan. 2021, influencermarketinghub.com/what-is-a-side-hustle/. Accessed 20 Feb. 2022.

"Side Hustle Meaning: What Is a Side Hustle, and Are They Worth It? [2022]." *Freelancing.school*, 2022, freelancing.school/side-hustle-meaning/.

Siders, Author Rose. "How to Be Successful in Your Side Hustle." *An Exercise in Frugality*, 30 July 2017, anexerciseinfrugality.com/successful-side-hustle/. Accessed 20 Feb. 2022.

"The Goldilocks Rule: How to Stay Motivated in Life and Business." *James Clear*, 28 June 2016, jamesclear.com/goldilocks-rule.

"The Power of Intrinsic Motivation." *Psychology Today*, www.psychologytoday.com/us/blog/mind-brain-and-value/202101/the-power-intrinsic-motivation.

"What Is Growth Mentality and Why Must Students Strive for It?" *Parasworldschool.com*, parasworldschool.com/what-is-growth-mentality-and-why-must-students-strive-for-it/. Accessed 20 Feb. 2022.

"What Is the Growth Mentality and Why Does It Matter?" *Ingle Learn*, 29 June 2021, inglelearn.com/what-is-the-growth-mentality-and-why-does-it-matter/. Accessed 20 Feb. 2022.

Lifehacker.com, 2019, lifehacker.com/four-ways-to-figure-out-what-you-really-want-to-do-with-513095544.